YOUR KNOWLEDGE HAS VALUE

- We will publish your bachelor's and master's thesis, essays and papers

- Your own eBook and book - sold worldwide in all relevant shops

- Earn money with each sale

Upload your text at www.GRIN.com
and publish for free

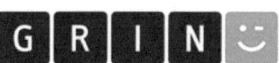

Bibliographic information published by the German National Library:

The German National Library lists this publication in the National Bibliography; detailed bibliographic data are available on the Internet at http://dnb.dnb.de .

This book is copyright material and must not be copied, reproduced, transferred, distributed, leased, licensed or publicly performed or used in any way except as specifically permitted in writing by the publishers, as allowed under the terms and conditions under which it was purchased or as strictly permitted by applicable copyright law. Any unauthorized distribution or use of this text may be a direct infringement of the author s and publisher s rights and those responsible may be liable in law accordingly.

Imprint:

Copyright © 2017 GRIN Verlag, Open Publishing GmbH
Print and binding: Books on Demand GmbH, Norderstedt Germany
ISBN: 9783668585300

This book at GRIN:

http://www.grin.com/en/e-book/381138/comprehensive-description-of-the-behavioral-approach-strengths-and-limitations

Patrick Kimuyu

Comprehensive Description of the Behavioral Approach. Strengths and Limitations of Behaviourism

GRIN Publishing

GRIN - Your knowledge has value

Since its foundation in 1998, GRIN has specialized in publishing academic texts by students, college teachers and other academics as e-book and printed book. The website www.grin.com is an ideal platform for presenting term papers, final papers, scientific essays, dissertations and specialist books.

Visit us on the internet:

http://www.grin.com/

http://www.facebook.com/grincom

http://www.twitter.com/grin_com

BEHAVIOURISM APPROACH: STREGTHS AND LIMITATIONS

Name: Patrick K. Kimuyu

It appears that the field of psychology is becoming extremely fascinating day-by-day owing to the sophistication of newly designed psychology approaches and research advancement. It is evidently true that the discipline of psychology has undergone transient evolution since its inception, and further developments are inevitable because; psychological research is currently widening to incorporate different perspective, which were not studied in psychology in the past. Initially, psychology emerged as one of the classical disciplines of science but, it has advanced significantly, especially after psychologists established the new branch of applied psychology whose application is gaining popularity. Currently, psychology does not only entail the social aspect of the human mind, but it also involves biological perspective and, this has led to the emergence of biopsychology and cognitive psychology.

Concisely, biopsychology applies biological and psychological approaches to investigate the interactions between the mind, behaviour, body and the environment and, it has expanded extensively in the field of psychoneuroimmunology and behavioural genetics (Mills College, 2013 par. 1). As such, it involves some of the most complex topics in biology such as genetics and the immune function in regard to the effects of environment on personality, mood and behaviour of an individual. In general, it deals with mechanisms through which the nervous system and the brain control behaviour. On the other hand, cognitive psychology deals mental processes, especially with regard to the information acquisition by the memory, processing and storage. As such, it studies all mental abilities ranging from perception, language processing to problem-solving in day-to-day life (Yale University, 2013 p. 1). However, it is worth noting that there are different approaches of psychology but, behaviourist approach seems to explain the interaction of the human mind and the environment. Therefore, this essay will provide a comprehensive description of the behavioural approach and evaluate its strengths and limitations.

Behaviourism is relatively different from the other psychology approaches, which focus on the functioning of the human brain in respect to emotion and thinking because; it is concerned primarily with the observable behaviour rather than the internal events. It entails the interpretation of human behaviour from the external events with regard to the environment. As such, it applies scientific and objective approaches to measure observable behaviour, which is usually interplay between biological functions of the brain and the environmental stimuli. Sammons remarks "show that people are quite capable of observing and learning from the behaviour and experiences of others" (p. 2). It is believed that behaviourism emerged as one of the principal paradigms of psychology during the first half of the 20th century, in which several assumptions on behavioural analysis and methodology formed a new avenue of understanding among psychologists. In behaviourism, individuals are believed to possess no free will in nature but, the interaction with the environment determines their observable behaviour (McLeod, 2007 p. 1). It is the stimulus-response association that is manifested as an individual's behaviour but, not necessarily the internal processes of the human brain. Therefore, behaviourism approach accomplishes one of the most fundamental purposes of psychology of predicting the outcome of a stimulus. McLeod (2007) reaffirms Watson's remarks, "the purpose of psychology [is] to predict, given the stimulus, what reaction will take place; or, given the reaction, state what the situation or stimulus is that has caused the reaction" (p. 1).

In regard to the evaluation of the behaviourism approach, this approach gains its strengths from the methodologies, which are adopted by behaviourists because; they involve significant insistence on precise measurements, control over variables and objectivity. This probably the reason as to why behaviourists are considered to have played significant roles in introducing behaviourism, which is a scientific method, into psychology (Sammons, n.d. p. 2). However, it is believed that this approach encompasses a number of drawbacks because; it applies methods, which study behaviour under artificial conditions or the so-called 'built environments'. In most cases, these artificial conditions have been evaluated to be relatively different from the real-world context and, this has attracted an unprecedented criticism, especially with regard to the use of animals in behavioural studies (Sammons, n.d. 2). Moreover, this approach is extensively criticised because it tends to overlook the significant influences of the internal mental processes associated with learning. The principle notion among behaviourists is that learning is attributable to personal experiences but, not the cognitive activity of the human brain; thus, behaviour is acquired. This understanding among behaviourists has been discredited after a comprehensive evaluation of some of its key theories such as classical and operant conditioning, in which the problem-solving ability of human beings is not adequately explained because the aspect of mental processes is excluded in studying human behaviour.

Strengths of behavioural approach are quite numerous compared to the other psychology approaches and this makes it one of the most viable approaches for studying human behaviour. Some of the most significant strengths of the behaviourism approach include its dependence on science, high applicability, a wide array of supportive experiments and its emphasis on objective measurements. In addition, behaviourism applies identified comparison between humans and animals in the interpretation of stimuli responses.

It is believed that the scientific approach of behaviourism enables behaviourists to study human behaviour through the use of controlled variables under objective measurements to establish the underlying effects and causes of the independent, extraneous and dependent variables. Precision in behaviourism can be attributed to a number of scientific features such as objectivity, control, hypothesis testing, predictability and replication. Control of variables enables behaviourists to establish the effect of dependent variables, whereas the cause of the stimulus is evaluated by the use of independent variables and, this enhances predictability of the future behaviour of an individual or experimental animal. On the other hand, scientific investigations are aimed at testing the hypothesis derived from a given theory; thus, experimental findings can be replicated to build a universal consensus among the experimentalists (McLeod, 2008 p. 2). As a result, the results obtained provide substantial evidence of the dramatic discoveries to avoid ambiguity as it is the case with the other psychology approaches.

The second strength of the behaviourism approach is that it is highly applicable. Some of the areas where behaviourism is applied include gender role development, behaviour modification, behavioural therapy, moral development, addiction to drugs and aggression. It is also applied in aversion therapy, language development, relationships and scientific methods (McLeod, 2007 p. 3). Its applicability has made it be highly accepted by experimentalists in psychology and other scientific disciplines leading to the advancement of research on human behaviour.

Thirdly, behaviourism approach involves numerous experiments, which provide supportive evidence to the theories applied in behavioural study in artificial conditions. This aspect has contributed significantly to the widespread popularity of the application of behaviourism approach in psychology and other scientific studies, which investigate human behaviour.

The fourth strength of the behaviourism approach is that it involves objective measurements, which enable experimentalists to avoid bias in behavioural findings. In behaviourism findings, behaviourists are ought to maintain the principal precepts of the research method; thus, they do not incorporate personal feelings and experiences in their studies. McLeod

(2008) states, "Researchers should remain totally value free when studying; they should try to remain totally unbiased in their investigations; researchers are not influenced by personal feelings and experiences" (p. 2). Therefore, objectivity minimizes bias in the research process while eliminating subjective ideas, which may lead to inappropriate interpretations of research results. The adoption of experimental objectivity enables investigators to obtain factual research outcomes even when the results do not match the expected outcomes. In other words, objectivity in behaviourism experiments enhances the unravelling of facts, rather than mere assumptions without substantial proof through documentation.

Moreover, behaviourism approach involves identified comparison between humans and animals for efficient interpretation of experimental data. Experiments in animal construct the foundation for behavioural studies in humans. For instance, Pavloc experimented classical conditioning with dogs and gained valuable insight, which prompted him to investigate the situation among humans. It is worth noting that, behaviourism is based on Pavloc's experiments, in the late 19th century. Other animals, which are extensively used in behaviourism studies are cats and rats, although some experiments involve humans from the beginning to the end of the experiments.

However, it is worth noting that behaviourism approach of psychology has got its limitations, despite the numerous strengths. The first limitation of this approach is that, it is extremely deterministic; thus, it gives little free-will to the investigators because; its experiments are conducted in hypothetical manner, and the outcomes are pre-determined. Investigators are supposed to stick to the outlined procedure and avoid personal attitudes as much as possible for universality of the experimental procedure. In behaviourism approach, the investigation procedures adopted by different behaviourists are expected to be homogeneous in nature to maintain replication of research approaches with different conditions and experimental animals.

Secondly, the behaviourism approach seems to ignore the core precepts of biology such as the influence of hormones and neurotransmitters, which are known to play pivotal roles in influencing an individual's behaviour. For instance, testosterone imparts maleness in men leading to the feeling of superiority but, this significant aspect is not considered in behaviourism; instead, behaviourists hold the notion that an individual's behaviour is learned through conditioning.

The third limitation of the behaviourism approach is that it involves low ecological validity because; it is based on experiments, which are usually conducted in artificial environments. In behaviourism, experimental animals are hardly exposed to the natural ecological conditions such as interaction with other animals and the ambient abiotic factors. It is believed that real-life experiences in the natural ecological conditions play a significant role in determining an individual's behaviour, and this can be evidenced with the impact of trauma caused by domestic violence on the behaviour of the children.

Fourthly, behaviourism approach encompasses humanism; thus, most psychologists reject the use of animals in experiments in essence that behavioural features can be investigated in artificial environments. They argue that, humans cannot be compared to animals. Moreover, behaviourism approach seems to ignore meditational processes, which are involved in the cognitive processes of the human mind, especially with regard to memory, problem-solving, thinking and learning (McLeod, 2007 p. 3).

On the other hand, there are some ethical issues relating to psychological research in behavioural approach, which tend to control its application. One of the most significant ethical issues is the fundamental conflict, which arises occasionally between the welfare of research participants and search for knowledge (Kimmel, 2007 p. 264). As a result, investigators are supposed to conduct their investigations in consideration of outlined guidelines, although in some circumstances, there is an unprecedented disagreement among researchers on the manner in which ethical decisions should be designed. Some of the ethical issues, which must be considered by investigators who involve human participants, include informed consent, deception, confidentiality, coercion to participate, invasion of privacy and potential psychological or physical harm on the participant (Pearson Education, 2010 p. 1). Other ethical issues include scientific misconduct and unethical behaviour, especially with regard to the misuse of power and sexual harassment of the participants.

In a brief conclusion, psychology has experienced extensive expansion, especially with regard to applied psychology leading to its popularity in the current world. However, it is worth noting that its rapid development can be attributed to some of its approaches such as the behaviourism approach, which has gained an unprecedented widespread application in most scientific fields such as biopsychology and cognitive psychology, which investigate the principal functions of the human brain. This approach is believed to have gained popularity because of its numerous strengths, which involve objectivity and reproducibility. However, it has several drawbacks, especially with regard to the ethical issues related to the approach although federal governments and professional organizations have addressed the issues by designing reliable regulations to guide investigators in experiments involving human participants.

References

Kimmel, A., 2007, *Ethical Issues in Behavioural Research: Basic and Applied Perspectives*, Hoboken, NJ: Wiley & Sons Inc.

McLeod, S., 2007, *Behaviourist Approach*, viewed 2 May, 2013, http://www.simplypsychology.org/behaviorism.html

McLeod, S., 2008, *Psychology as a Science*, viewed 2 May, 2013, http://www.simplypsychology.org/science-psychology.html

Mills College, 2013, *Biopsychology*, viewed 2 May, 2013, http://www.mills.edu/academics/undergraduate/biopsyc/

Pearson Education (2010). *Ethical Issues in Behavioural Research*, viewed 3 May, 2013, http://wps.ablongman.com/ab_leary_resmethod_4/11/2990/765554.cw/index.html

Sammons, A., n.d., *The behaviourist approach: the basics*, viewed 3 May, 2013, http://www.psychlotron.org.uk/newResources/approaches/AS_AQB_approaches_BehaviourismBasics.pdf

Yale University, 2013, *Cognitive Psychology*, viewed 2 May, 2013, http://psychology.yale.edu/research_area/cognitive-psychology

YOUR KNOWLEDGE HAS VALUE

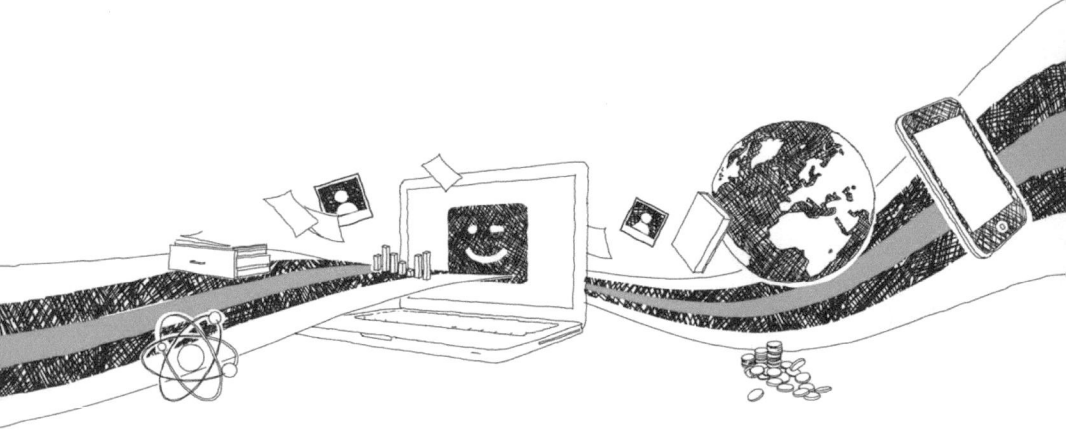

- We will publish your bachelor's and master's thesis, essays and papers

- Your own eBook and book - sold worldwide in all relevant shops

- Earn money with each sale

Upload your text at www.GRIN.com
and publish for free